Keto for 2

Simple and Mouthwatering Ketogenic Diet Recipes For Two People

Faith Smith

About The Author

For most of my life, I did not have to worry too much about my weight; I was not the fittest person but I was also not overweight, which was good enough for me. However, after I gave birth to my lovely son, things changed; I gained quite a bit of weight and I did not exactly like what I saw. I was not as confident as I once was and I was very conscious of how I looked and how the clothes I wore made me look. Once my son turned one and was not breastfeeding as much, I started researching for ways to lose weight.

In my quest to lose weight, I have tried quite a bit of different things from the ketogenic diet and intermittent fasting to smoothie cleanses. Since all these have worked for me, I have incorporated them into my lifestyle and I must say, so far I like what I see.

I understand how difficult losing weight can be and to make it easier for you, I write books on what has worked for me and how you can lose weight to achieve your desired body.

I have still not achieved my dream body but I am happy with the progress so far and that is good enough because life is not perfect and I am okay with good enough.

This document is geared towards providing exact and reliable information in regards to the topic and issue covered. The publication is sold with the idea that the publisher is not required to render accounting, officially permitted, or otherwise, qualified services. If advice is necessary, legal or professional, a practiced individual in the profession should be ordered.

- From a Declaration of Principles which was accepted and approved equally by a Committee of the American Bar Association and a Committee of Publishers and Associations.

In no way is it legal to reproduce, duplicate, or transmit any part of this document in either electronic means or in printed format. Recording of this publication is strictly prohibited and any storage of this document is not allowed unless with written permission from the publisher. All rights reserved.

The information provided herein is stated to be truthful and consistent, in that any liability, in terms of inattention or otherwise, by any usage or abuse of any policies, processes, or directions contained within is the solitary and utter responsibility of the recipient reader. Under no circumstances will any legal responsibility or blame be held against the publisher for any reparation, damages, or monetary loss due to the information herein, either directly or indirectly.

Respective authors own all copyrights not held by the publisher.

The information herein is offered for informational purposes solely, and is universal as so. The presentation of the information is without contract or any type of guarantee assurance.

The trademarks that are used are without any consent, and the publication of the trademark is without permission or backing by the trademark owner. All trademarks and brands within this book are for clarifying purposes only and are the owned by the owners themselves, not affiliated with this document.

Table of Contents

Introduction

By now I believe you have heard great things about the ketogenic diet and are excited to get started with the diet. The keto diet is simply a low-carb, high-fat diet that seeks to get your body into a metabolic state known as ketosis where you burn fat for energy.

In addition to weight loss, the ketogenic diet offers a variety of benefits such as:

- Increased energy

- Better management of diabetes

- Reduced risk of suffering from cardiovascular diseases

- Greater mental clarity

In order to ensure your success with this diet, you need to just eat until you are full or you will undo the great results. The amazing thing is the keto diet requires you to eat more fat and leafy green vegetables, which are both quite filing; therefore, you are assured of getting full. If you have a difficult time with portion control, this book is for you as it provides simple recipes with only 2 servings.

Let us get started with some breakfast recipes:

Chapter 1: Breakfast Recipes

Baked Green Eggs

Servings: 2

Ingredients

4 medium eggs

1 tablespoon finely grated gruyere (you can use a vegetarian alternative)

100ml double cream

4 tablespoons fresh pesto

100g baby spinach, roughly chopped

Directions

1. Preheat the oven to 180 degrees C for gas or 200 degrees C for fan.

2. In a bowl, mix the pesto, spinach, seasoning and cream. Once done divide the mixture into 2 shallow oven-safe dishes. Sprinkle some cheese over each of the portions.

3. In each portion, create a shallow hollow and then break two eggs into each hole. Bake the mixture for 10-12

minutes. The egg whites should be set and the yolks still runny.

4. Once the eggs are ready, carefully remove from the oven and serve.

Nutritional information per serving: Calories 579, Fat 54g, Protein 19g, Carbs 3g

Spinach Avocado Smoothie

Servings: 2

Ingredients

Sweetener, to taste

2 teaspoons vanilla extract

1 ripe avocado, deseeded

1 cup coconut milk (unsweetened – from refrigerated cartons, not cans)

2 cups spinach (or other leafy greens)

Directions

1. Into a blender, add the ingredients and pulse until smooth.

2. Serve and enjoy.

Nutritional information per serving: Calories 190, Fat 17g, Protein 3g, Carbs 10g

Keto Toast

Servings: 2

Ingredients

2 1/2 tablespoons ghee, melted

1 egg, whisked

1/8 teaspoon salt

1/2 teaspoon baking powder

1/3 cup almond flour

Directions

1. Preheat the oven to 200 C (400 F).

2. Into a mug, add the ingredients and stir to combine.

3. Microwave for 90 seconds on high.

4. Once done, allow the bread to cool and then carefully remove it from the mug and then slice it into 4 slices.

5. Arrange the four slices on a baking tray and then place them in the oven and toast for 4 minutes.

6. Enjoy. You can spread a little ghee on top if you wish and make a sandwich with eggs and bacon.

Nutritional information per serving: Calories 270, Fat 27g, Protein 6g, Carbs 3g

Egg Avocado

Servings: 2

Ingredients

1 tablespoon chopped chives

1/8 teaspoon pepper

4 fresh eggs

2 ripe avocados

Directions

1. Preheat the oven to 425 degrees F.

2. Slice the 2 avocados in half lengthwise. Get rid of the pit and then scoop out a bit of flesh from the avocado. You can scoop out 2 tablespoons. The egg should be able to fit well in the center.

3. In a small baking dish, arrange the avocados and then crack an egg into each avocado half.

4. Bake for 15-20 minutes. The eggs whites need to set.

5. Remove from the oven. Season with chives and pepper and serve. You can serve with your favorite garnish if you wish.

Nutritional information per serving: Calories 449, Fat 38.2g, Protein 15.2g, Carbs 18.1g

Tomato and Eggs

Servings: 2

Ingredients

Sea salt & cracked black pepper to taste

1 teaspoon fresh Italian parsley

2 large eggs

2 medium/large fresh tomatoes

Directions

1. Preheat the oven to 350 degrees F.

2. Line the baking sheet using aluminum foil.

3. Carefully chop the tops off the tomatoes and then use a spoon to scoop out the fleshy innards.

4. Once done, crack an egg into each well and then bake for 30 minutes

5. Allow to cool and then garnish with salt, pepper and minced parsley.

6. Serve and enjoy.

Nutritional information per serving: Calories 186, Fat 10g, Protein 14g, Carbs 6g

Avocado and Bacon

Servings: 2

Ingredients

¼ teaspoon sea salt

2 large pastured, organic eggs

1 large avocado, peeled and cut in slices

4 strips of uncured, pastured bacon

Directions

1. Place a ceramic pan over medium heat and then add the bacon and avocado slices. Cook for about 3 minutes and then flip to cook the other side.

2. Once done, remove the bacon and avocado and set aside. Make sure you keep them warm.

3. In the same frying pan, crack the eggs and fry them for 2-3 minutes. Flip the eggs, and cook to desired consistency.

4. Remove and serve with the bacon and avocado.

5. Enjoy.

Nutritional information per serving: Calories 313, Fat 26g, Protein 13g, Carbs 2.5g

Kale and Sausage Crumb

Servings: 2

Ingredients

1/2 medium avocado

Fresh herbs such as parsley

Optional: 1/2 teaspoon paprika or chilli

Salt and pepper to taste

1 tablespoon of butter, ghee or duck fat

1 cup chopped kale

2-3 good quality gluten-free sausages

1 teaspoon extra virgin olive oil or ghee

4 large eggs

Directions

1. Skin the sausages carefully and then discard the skin. In a pan, heat up 1 tablespoon of the olive oil. Once done, cook the sausage meat for about 10 minutes. Use a wooden spoon or spatula to break up the sausage as it cooks. The sausage meat should resemble a crumb.

2. Add the kale and the paprika or chili and cook for 1 minute and then set aside.

3. In a cup, crack the eggs and then season with salt and pepper. Whisk well using a fork. Scramble the beaten eggs for about 1 minute. Use a wooden spoon to scramble in order to prevent sticking.

4. Remove from the heat and let the eggs firm up and then divide between two plates.

5. Top each plate with the avocado, sausage crumb and some fresh herbs.

6. Serve immediately.

Nutritional information per serving: Calories 529, Fat 42.7g, Protein 30.4g, Carbs 6.6g

Keto Almond Porridge

Servings: 2

Ingredients

1/2 cup almonds, ground using a blender or food processor

Dash of nutmeg, cloves and cardamom

1 teaspoon cinnamon powder

Stevia to taste (optional)

3/4 cup coconut milk

Directions

1. In a small saucepan over medium heat, heat up the coconut milk.

2. Add in the sweetener and ground almonds and stir for about 5 minutes. The mixture should thicken a bit more.

3. Stir in the spices. You can add more spices or sweetener if need be. Add a bit at a time to gauge the taste and adjust if necessary.

4. Remove and serve hot.

Nutritional information per serving: Calories 294, Fat 29g, Protein 6g, Carbs 8g

Coconut Flour Porridge

Servings: 2

Ingredients

Toppings:

60 grams blueberries

2 tablespoons butter

Porridge:

1 pinch salt

10 drops liquid stevia

1 teaspoon vanilla extract

1 teaspoon cinnamon

1/4 cup coconut flour

1/4 cup ground flaxseed

1 cup almond milk

Directions

1. In a saucepan, heat up the almond milk over a low flame.

2. Add the coconut flour, cinnamon, flaxseed and salt and whisk together to break up the clumps.

3. Heat the mixture until slightly bubbling. Once bubbling, add in the vanilla extract and liquid stevia and stir to incorporate.

4. When the porridge reaches your desired consistency, turn the flame off and top with your favorite toppings.

5. Serve immediately.

Nutritional information per serving: Calories 405, Fat 34g, Protein 10g, Carbs 8g

Pecan Porridge

Servings: 2

Ingredients

1/2 teaspoon cinnamon

1/4 cup unsweetened toasted coconut

1/4 cup chopped pecans or walnuts

2 tablespoons hemp seeds

2 tablespoons chia seeds

1 tablespoon extra-virgin coconut oil

1/4 cup almond butter

3/4 cup unsweetened almond milk

1/4 cup coconut milk

Optional: 5-10 drops liquid stevia (NuNaturals or SweetLeaf)

Directions

1. In a small saucepan, combine the almond milk, coconut milk and almond butter. Bring the mixture to a simmer over medium-heat.

2. Once the mixture is heated through, remove the saucepan from the heat.

3. Add the hemp seeds, toasted coconut, chia seeds and chopped pecans.

4. Add the stevia and cinnamon and stir well. Allow the mixture to sit for 5-10 minutes.

5. Serve the porridge in bowls, top with some pecans and serve. You can serve hot or cold if you wish.

Nutritional information per serving: Calories 582, Fat 51.7g, Protein 13.8g, Carbs 5.2g

Keto Oatmeal

Servings: 2

Ingredients

5-10 drops Stevia extract

1 cup water

1/2 cup coconut milk

1 teaspoon vanilla extract

1/3 cup flaked almonds

1/3 cup flaked coconut

1/4 cup shredded coconut

1/4 cup Chia Seeds

Directions

1. In a frying pan, carefully brown the flaked almonds and flaked coconut for 2 minutes.

2. Once done, place all the ingredients in a saucepan over medium heat. Cook on medium-high heat for 7-10 minutes ensuring that you stir well every 30 seconds.

3. Remove and serve hot.

Nutritional information per serving: Calories 314, Fat 23g, Protein 11g, Carbs 1 g

Keto Porridge

Servings: 2

Ingredients

1-2 teaspoons monk fruit sweetener, optional

1 teaspoon vanilla, optional

1/2 tablespoon ground cinnamon, optional

1/3 cup canned full fat coconut milk

1/2 cup water

1 tablespoon coconut flour

1/4 cup hemp seeds

1/2 cup flaked unsweetened coconut

Directions

1. Add the hemp seeds, coconut, milk and water into a medium saucepan,.

2. Bring the ingredients to a simmer for about 2 minutes. The porridge should thicken.

3. Add the cinnamon and vanilla and stir to combine.

4. Remove and serve. You can serve with more milk and your favorite toppings.

Nutritional information per serving: Calories 374, Fat 33g, Protein 11g, Carbs 9g

Almond Flour Waffles

Servings: 2

Ingredients

1/2 teaspoon vanilla extract

1/4 cup unsweetened almond milk

2 tablespoons butter

2 tablespoons almond butter

1/4 teaspoon sea salt

1/2 teaspoon gluten-free baking powder

2 tablespoons erythritol (or any sweetener)

1/2 cup blanched almond flour

1 large egg (separated)

Directions

1. Preheat your waffle iron to high. Grease the waffle iron lightly using oil spray.

2. In the meantime, put the egg white into a medium bowl and then beat it to stiff peaks. Once done, set aside.

3. In a bowl, mix the almond flour, baking powder, salt and erythritol and set aside.

4. In a microwave-safe small bowl, melt the almond butter and butter. Once done, whisk well and then add the mixture into the dry flour in the bowl.

5. Add the vanilla, almond milk and yolk and mix with the batter until smooth.

6. Gently fold the egg whites in and mix well to incorporate. Don't over mix. The batter should be fluffy and light.

7. Once done, place half the butter into the prepared waffle iron. Close the waffle iron and cook for about 5 minutes. Turn off the waffle iron and allow it to cool a bit before removing the waffle. Cook the remaining batter.

Nutritional information per serving: Calories 401, Fat 37g, Protein 13g, Carbs 9g

Overnight "Oats"

Servings: 2

Ingredients

2/3 cup full-fat coconut milk, plus more for serving

1/2 cup Hemp Hearts

1 tablespoon chia seeds

3-4 drops of liquid stevia

1/2 teaspoon vanilla extract

Pinch of finely ground Himalayan rock salt

6 whole raspberries, optional toppings

Sliced almonds, optional toppings

Directions

1. Add all the ingredients into a mason jar and stir to mix. Put in the fridge for at least 8 hours. You can leave it overnight if you wish.

2. In the morning, add some milk to your desired consistency and divide the meal between two bowls.

3. Top with raspberries and whole almonds and serve.

4. Enjoy. You can store the "oatmeal" in the fridge for up to 2 days if you wish. Place it in an airtight container before storing.

Nutritional information per serving: Calories 408, Fat 34.7g, Protein 15.3g, Carbs 9.1g

Chapter 2: Lunch Recipes

Avocado Tuna Salad

Servings: 2

Ingredients

2 tablespoons chopped fresh dill

1/2 teaspoon pepper

1/2 teaspoon salt

1 teaspoon lemon zest

2 teaspoons lemon juice

1/2 cup finely chopped celery

1 medium avocado

2 pouches extra virgin oil Yellowfin Tuna

Directions

1. In a bowl, combine all the ingredients. You can use a fork to mash the avocado so as to incorporate it well.

2. Once done, use foil to cover the bowl and chill in the refrigerator for 1-2 hours.

3. Serve and enjoy.

Nutritional information per serving: Calories 368, Fat 27.4g, Protein 21.6g, Carbs 13.2g

Keto Egg Salad

Servings: 2

Ingredients

1/2 tablespoon fresh chopped parsley (optional)

1/8 teaspoon dill (optional)

Splash of lemon juice

1 teaspoon Dijon mustard

1/3 cup mayonnaise

6 eggs

1 avocado

Salt and pepper, to taste

Directions

1. Place the eggs in a saucepan and then cover them with water. Bring the water to a boil. Turn the heat off and cover the saucepan. Allow the eggs to rest in the boiled water for about 10-15 minutes.

2. Once the time elapses, run the eggs under running cold water and then carefully peel the shells.

3. Slice the eggs into bite-sized pieces and then sprinkle some salt and pepper on top and set aside.

4. Use a fork to mash the avocado and then mix in some salt and pepper to taste.

5. In a medium bowl, combine the eggs, mustard, mayo, mashed avocado, herbs and lemon juice. Chill the mixture in the refrigerator.

6. Serve and enjoy.

Nutritional information per serving: Calories 575, Fat 51g, Protein 20g, Carbs 7g

Keto Salmon Curry

Servings: 2

Ingredients

2 tablespoons coconut oil, to cook with

1 lb. of raw salmon, diced, defrosted

2 cups bone broth

Cream from the top of 1 (14-oz) can of coconut milk

1 teaspoon garlic powder

1 ½ tablespoons curry powder

2 cups green beans, diced

1/2 medium onion, diced or finely chopped

2 tablespoons basil, chopped, for garnish

Salt and pepper, to taste

Directions

1. In a saucepan, heat the coconut oil and sauté the diced onion until translucent.

2. Add the green beans and cook for several minutes.

3. Add the water or broth and bring the ingredients to a boil.

4. Add the garlic powder, salmon and curry powder, and stir.

5. Add in the coconut cream and simmer for 3-5 minutes. The salmon should be cooked through.

6. Season with some salt and pepper.

7. Once done, top with chopped basil and serve.

Nutritional information per serving: Calories 640, Fat 44g, Protein 49g, Carbs 16g

Spring Soup with Egg

Servings: 2

Ingredients

Salt to taste

1 head of romaine lettuce, chopped

32 oz. chicken broth

2 eggs

Directions

1. Put the chicken broth in a pot over high heat, and bring it to a boil.

2. Once the broth has boiled, reduce the heat and poach the eggs inside the broth for about 5 minutes. The eggs should be a bit runny.

3. Carefully remove the eggs and put one in each bowl.

4. Into the pot, add the chopped romaine and stir it into the broth. Cook for several minutes until wilted.

5. Add the broth into the bowls of poached eggs and serve.

Nutritional information per serving: Calories 150, Fat 5g, Protein 16g, Carbs 11g

Coconut Curry

Servings: 2

Ingredients

½ cup coconut cream

1 tablespoon red curry paste

2 teaspoons soy sauce

2 teaspoons Fysh sauce

1 teaspoon minced ginger

1 teaspoon minced garlic

¼ medium onion

4 tablespoons coconut oil

1 large handful of spinach

1 cup broccoli florets

Directions

1. Into a pan, add 2 tablespoons of the coconut oil and then heat it over medium-high heat.

2. In the meantime, mince the garlic and slice the onions. Once the oil is hot, sauté the onion. Allow them to sizzle, and cook for 3-4 minutes or until semi-translucent and caramelized.

3. Add the garlic and cook for 30 seconds. It should brown slightly.

4. Set the heat to medium-low. Into the pan, add the broccoli florets and stir well. Cook for 1-2 minutes to allow the flavors to mix.

5. Carefully move the ingredients in the pan to one side and then spread 1 tablespoon of the red curry paste at the bottom of the cleared side and cook for a few minutes then stir to mix with the other ingredients.

6. Spread a handful of spinach on top of the ingredients and allow the spinach to wilt.

7. Add the coconut cream and stir to combine.

8. Add 2 teaspoons of the Fysh sauce, 2 tablespoons of coconut oil, 1 teaspoon of minced ginger and 2 teaspoons of soy sauce and mix well. Simmer the mixture for 5-10 minutes. The longer you simmer, the thicker the sauce will be.

9. Turn off the heat and serve. You can garnish with black sesame seeds and red cabbage if you wish.

Nutritional information per serving: Calories 398, Fat 40.73g, Protein 3.91g, Carbs 7.86g

Zucchini and Avocado Pesto

Servings: 2

Ingredients

5-6 leaves fresh basil, to garnish

1 tablespoon olive oil

Optional: Italian seasoning

Salt and pepper to taste

Avocado Walnut Pesto:

½ cup water, if needed

¼ cup Parmesan cheese, grated

½ large lemon

2 cloves garlic, peeled

¼ cup walnuts

1 cup fresh basil leaves

½ large avocado

Zucchini Ribbons:

½ teaspoon salt

3 medium zucchini

Directions

1. Use a mandolin slicer or vegetable peeler to carefully slice the zucchini into thin ribbons.

2. Into a colander, add the zucchini slices and a bit of salt and toss to combine. Let the zucchini stand for a bit as you make the pesto.

3. Add the avocado pesto ingredients to a food processor. Blend the ingredients to make a smooth sauce. You can thin out the sauce by adding a bit of water if need be.

4. Use 1 tablespoon of olive oil to carefully grease a skillet over medium heat.

5. Add the zucchini slices and cook for 3-5 minutes. They should just begin to soften. Once done, remove the slices from the heat.

6. Pour the pesto on top of the zucchini slices and toss well to coat.

7. Divide into 2 portions and then garnish with grated parmesan and fresh basil.

8. Enjoy.

Nutritional information per serving: Calories 325.5, Fat 26.08g, Protein 10.65g, Carbs 18.01g

Vegetables and Goat Cheese Salad

Servings: 2

Ingredients

1 tablespoon avocado oil

4 cups arugula, divided between two bowls

½ cup baby Portobello mushrooms, sliced

1 medium red bell pepper, seeds removed & cut into 8 pieces

4 ounces goat cheese, cut into 4 ½ in thick medallions

1 teaspoon garlic flakes

1 teaspoon onion flakes

2 tablespoons sesame seeds

2 tablespoons poppy seeds

Directions

1. In a small dish, combine the sesame seeds, poppy seeds, garlic flakes and onion.

2. Coat the pieces of goat cheese well on both sides and then place them on a plate and refrigerate until ready to fry.

50

3. Coat a nonstick skillet with spray and place it on medium heat. Cook the mushrooms and peppers until both sides are slightly charred. The peppers should soften. Divide the mushrooms and peppers into the two bowls of arugula.

4. Into the skillet, add the goat cheese and fry for 30 seconds on each side. Be sure to flip gently as the cheese tends to melt quickly.

5. Add the cheese to each bowl of salad and then drizzle some avocado oil on top.

6. Serve warm.

Nutritional information per serving: Calories 350, Fat 27.61g, Protein 16.09g, Carbs 12.28g

Mushroom Pasta

Servings: 2

Ingredients

3/4 tub thick cream

Pinch of dried parsley

1 teaspoon almond flour

3 cups assorted mushrooms

2 cloves garlic

2 tablespoons butter

2 packs shirataki noodles

Fresh parsley finely chopped, to garnish

Olive oil

1/4 teaspoon pepper

1/4 teaspoon salt

Directions

1. In a frying pan, dry fry the shirataki noodles until you hear a whistling sound. The sound lets you know that the

52

excess moisture is being expelled from the noodles. Once done, set aside.

2. Into the frying pan, add some butter and the cook the garlic for 1 minute.

3. Stir in the mushrooms and coat with the garlic and oil. Sauté for 5 minutes as you stir occasionally. The mushrooms should turn a golden color. Once done, remove the mushrooms but leave the drippings behind.

4. Into the drippings, add the dried parsley, almond flour and cream. Stir well.

5. Stir in the salt and pepper and cook for a few more minutes.

6. Return the shirataki and mushrooms to the frying pan and stir to combine.

7. Serve hot. You can garnish with fresh parsley if you wish.

Nutritional information per serving: Calories 237, Fat 20g, Protein 6g, Carbs 14g

Chicken and Avocado Salad

Servings: 2

Ingredients

25g pumpkin seeds

1 avocado

20g rocket leaves

100g little gem lettuce leaves

Freshly ground black pepper

Fine Himalayan pink salt

⅛ teaspoon paprika

2 teaspoons apple cider vinegar

1 tablespoon Dijon mustard

1 handful fresh tarragon leaves

½ lemon (juice only)

150g Greek yoghurt

6 rashers of bacon (or 180g raw pancetta slices)

400g chicken (cooked and cut into 7-8cm strips)

Directions

1. Prepare the dressing. Start by mixing the lemon juice, yogurt, apple cider vinegar, Dijon mustard, chopped tarragon and paprika. Add some salt and pepper according to taste.

2. Add the chicken to the dressing and stir well to coat. If you are not using pre-cooked chicken, first pan-fry the chicken in some olive oil and season it well and add some herbs before mixing it with the dressing.

3. Once done, cover the bowl using cling film and then allow the chicken to marinate for at least 2 hours in the refrigerator. You can refrigerate overnight if you want.

4. Cook the pancetta or bacon until crispy. Once done, set on top of paper towels and allow it to cool. Once cooled, slice into pieces.

5. Slice the avocado and toast the pumpkin seeds.

6. Assemble the salad. Divide the lettuce leaves into two plates and then add the rocket leaves. Add the chicken and then top with the bacon slices and avocado slices.

7. Garnish with the pumpkin seeds and then serve.

Nutritional information per serving: Calories 812, Fat 46g, Protein 81g, Carbs 8g

Chapter 3: Dinner Recipes

Keto Chicken

Servings: 2

Ingredients

100g creme fraiche

1.5 tablespoons chopped, fresh parsley

3 tablespoons chopped, fresh coriander

¼ teaspoon coriander powder

A sprinkle of freshly ground black pepper

¼ teaspoon chili powder

1 teaspoon paprika powder

¼ teaspoon ground cumin

½ teaspoon fine Himalayan pink salt

2 garlic cloves (minced)

1 lemon

2 tablespoons MCT oil or flaxseed oil

2 tablespoons extra virgin olive oil (EVOO)

8 boneless skinless chicken thighs

Directions

1. In a zip lock bag, add the ground cumin, black pepper, paprika powder, coriander powder, salt and chili powder and then shake the bag well. Set this aside.

2. In another bag, add the chicken, minced garlic, 1 tablespoon of chopped parsley, grated lemon zest plus the juice of half a lemon, 2 tablespoons chopped coriander and the extra virgin olive oil.

3. Once done, gently massage the chicken. Make sure it is well coated and then carefully squeeze out the air from the zip lock bag. Seal the bag.

4. Allow the chicken to marinate overnight in the refrigerator.

5. On the next day, let the chicken sit at room temperature for one hour.

6. Once the time is up, grill the chicken for 5 minutes per side.

7. Drizzle the flaxseed or MCT oil on top and then top with coriander leaves. Serve the chicken with the coriander dip.

8. Enjoy.

Nutritional information per serving: Calories 736, Fat 58g, Protein 51g, Carbs 3g

Cajun Prawns

Servings: 2

Ingredients

¼ teaspoon fine Himalayan pink salt

1 garlic clove (minced)

½ teaspoon dried oregano

½ teaspoon dried thyme

¼ teaspoon chili powder

1 tablespoon sweet paprika

¼ teaspoon dried onion powder

⅛ teaspoon cayenne pepper

3 tablespoons extra virgin olive oil (EVOO)

700g Argentine prawns (about 24 shrimp)

Directions

1. Remove the shell from the prawns but leave the tails on.

2. Score along the dorsal length using a sharp knife. You should score it enough to expose the bowel. Once done, remove the bowel gently from each prawn.

3. Rinse the prawns in running water and then drain and set aside. You can place the prawns in a Pyrex bowl or a large glass bowl.

4. In a small bowl, mix the spices and seasoning.

5. Take the olive oil and pour it onto the prawns and then coat with the spices mixture. Stir well to coat evenly. Once done, use cling film to cover the Pyrex bowl and allow the prawns to marinate for a few hours in the fridge.

6. Coat a cast iron pan with a bit of EVOO and then set the heat to medium-high.

7. Sauté the prawns for 3-5 minutes per side. They should be slightly charred.

8. Serve immediately. You can serve with avocado salad if you wish.

Nutritional information per serving: Calories 528, Fat 31g, Protein 59g, Carbs 1.5g

Low Carb Meatza

Servings: 2

Ingredients

1 cup mozzarella cheese

¾ cup low-carb tomato sauce

¼ cup Parmesan cheese

1 teaspoon pepper

1 teaspoon garlic

1 teaspoon basil

1 teaspoon rosemary

1 teaspoon thyme

½ tablespoon oregano

1 large egg

12-ounce can chicken breast

Directions

1. Preheat the oven to 350 degrees F.

2. In a bowl, add the chicken and mash it up. Make sure it is very fine to avoid a chunky crust.

3. Into the bowl, add the egg, parmesan cheese and spices, and mix well. You can add more spices if you prefer a stronger flavor.

4. Place the mixture in your pizza pan and use a fork to push it down. Place the pizza in the oven and cook for 15 minutes. The top should brown a little.

5. Add the sauce and spread it evenly.

6. Spread the cheese on top and then bake for an additional 15 minutes.

7. Remove and serve.

Nutritional information per serving: Calories 446, Fat 25.52g, Protein 46.07g, Carbs 8.9g

Broccoli Soup

Servings: 2

Ingredients

1 cup water

2 small heads of broccoli chopped into florets

2 teaspoons fresh ginger chopped

1 teaspoon turmeric powder

1 teaspoon salt

1 can unsweetened coconut milk

3 cloves garlic

1 onion

Directions

1. Into a pan over low heat, add half of the coconut milk.

2. Add the garlic and onion and then cook until soft. This should take about 5 minutes.

3. Now add in the turmeric, ginger, salt, water, the rest of the coconut milk and the broccoli florets. Simmer the

ingredients for one hour while stirring occasionally and mash the broccoli.

4. When ready, let the mixture to cool a bit and then place it in your food processor. Pulse the soup into a puree. You can puree in small batches if need be.

5. Serve with fresh greens, roasted almonds, and yogurt and sesame seeds if you wish.

Nutritional information per serving: Calories 439, Fat 36g, Protein 8g, Carbs 17g

Keto Meatballs

Servings: 2

Ingredients

Creamy Tomato Sauce & Toppings:

1/4 teaspoon crushed red pepper flakes

2 tablespoons finely chopped fresh parsley

1/4 cup finely grated parmesan cheese

2 tablespoons heavy whipping cream

1 cup marinara sauce like Rao's

Meatballs:

1/2 teaspoon salt

1/2 teaspoon black pepper

1/2 teaspoon dried oregano

1/2 teaspoon garlic powder

1 teaspoon dry minced onion

1/2 cup marinara sauce like Rao's

1/2 cup finely grated parmesan cheese

1 large egg

1 pound 80% lean ground beef, patted dry

Directions

1. Preheat the oven to 350 degrees F. Prepare a 9 by 13 inch baking dish by lining it with parchment paper or foil. This will make for an easier cleanup.

2. Add the ingredients for the meatballs into a large bowl and mix well. Once done, form the mixture into 16 meatballs. The meatballs should be about 2 inches in diameter.

3. Carefully place the meatballs in the baking dish. They should not touch each other.

4. Bake for 25-30 minutes or until cooked through. The internal temperature should be 165F.

5. In the meantime, prepare the sauce. Start by simmering the marinara sauce for 5 minutes in a saucepan making sure that you stir frequently. Once done, set the heat to low. The sauce should form an orange hue.

6. Once the meatballs are cooked through, place them on the serving plates.

7. Top with the creamy sauce and parmesan cheese and then sprinkle the crushed red pepper and parsley on top.

8. Serve hot.

Nutritional information per serving: Calories 540, Fat 19g, Protein 75g, Carbs 8g

Creamy Mustard Pork Loin

Servings: 2

Ingredients

2 cups green beans, optional

Mustard Sauce:

1 tablespoon mustard

1/2 lemon

1 teaspoon apple cider vinegar

1/4 cup heavy cream

1/2 cup chicken broth

Pork Loins:

1 teaspoon thyme

1 teaspoon paprika

1 teaspoon black pepper

1 tablespoon pink Himalayan sea salt

4 4 oz. pork loins

Directions

1. Use a paper towel to pat your pork loins dry. Once done, season the pork loins with salt, paprika, thyme and pepper.

2. Place a large pan on high heat and sear the pork loins for 2-3 minutes per side and set aside.

3. Lower the flame and then prepare the sauce. Into the pan, add the apple cider vinegar, chicken broth and 1/4 cup of heavy cream. Allow the mixture to come to a simmer.

4. Once simmering, add a tablespoon of mustard and the juice from half a lemon; stir well to mix.

5. Return the pork loins to the pan and coat them well with the sauce after flipping them once. Cook for 10 minutes while slightly open

6. Once done, serve with sauce and green beans.

7. Enjoy.

Nutritional information per serving: Calories 480, Fat 30g, Protein 46g, Carbs 1g

Beef Wraps

Servings: 2

Ingredients

1 lb. ground beef

8 cabbage leaves

2 teaspoons cumin

4 clove garlic

1 teaspoon ginger

2 tablespoons cilantro

1 bell pepper

2/3 lbs. ground beef

1 onion

2 tablespoons coconut oil

Directions

1. Add the coconut oil into a frying pan over medium heat and sauté the onions. Add in the peppers and ground beef and cook.

2. Once the ground beef is cooked through, add the ginger, cilantro, cumin, garlic, salt and pepper.

3. In the meantime, add water to a large pot. It should be about 3/4 full. Place the cabbage leaves for 20 seconds in the boiling water and then plunge them in cold water. You can work with one leaf at a time. Once done, place the leaves on a plate.

4. Carefully add some beef mixture on each leaf and fold into a roll.

5. Enjoy.

Nutritional information per serving: Calories 375, Fat 26g, Protein 30g, Carbs 4g

Sesame Chicken

Servings: 2

Ingredients

Sesame Sauce:

1/4 teaspoon xanthan gum

2 tablespoons sesame seeds

1 clove garlic

Ginger (1 cm cube)

1 tablespoon vinegar

2 tablespoon Sukrin Gold

1 tablespoon toasted sesame seed oil

2 tablespoons soy sauce

Coating & Chicken:

Pepper

Salt

1 tablespoon toasted sesame seed oil

1 lb. chicken thighs (cut into bite sized pieces)

1 tablespoon arrowroot powder

1 egg

Directions

1. Into a mixing bowl, add the arrowroot powder and a large egg and whisk to combine.

2. Once done, add the bite sized chicken pieces and coat them well.

3. In a large pan, heat the tablespoon of toasted sesame oil. Once hot, add the chicken thighs and make sure there is some room in between the chicken thighs. You can work in two batches to avoid overcrowding. Cook for 10 minutes and be gentle as you flip the chicken pieces.

4. In the meantime, prepare the sesame sauce by combining the sauce ingredients and whisking well.

5. Once the chicken is cooked through, pour the sesame sauce on top and stir. Cook for 5 minutes to thicken the sauce.

6. Once the sauce is thick, serve the chicken with sautéed broccoli, green onions and more sesame seeds.

7. Enjoy.

Nutritional information per serving: Calories 520, Fat 36g, Protein 45g, Carbs 4g

Pork Chops and Cabbage

Servings: 2

Ingredients

The Cabbage:

Sea salt to taste

1/8 teaspoon red chili flakes

1/4 cup chicken broth

1 tablespoon apple cider vinegar

6 oz. cabbage sliced into strips

The Pork Chops:

1 teaspoon ghee

1/8 teaspoon sea salt

1/8 teaspoon garlic powder

1/8 teaspoon coriander ground

2 boneless pork chops

Directions

1. Use the garlic powder, coriander and sea salt to season both sides of the pork chops. Ensure you season the pork chops well.

2. Into a cast iron skillet, melt some ghee over medium heat. Once the ghee is melted, add the pork chops and cook them for about 4 to 5 minutes each side. They should reach the temperature of 160F for medium or 145F for medium rare. Once done, allow the pork chops to sit for 5 minutes before you slice them.

3. In another skillet over high heat, bring the cabbage, broth, chili flakes, vinegar and sea salt to a boil while stirring the ingredients occasionally. Continue cooking until the cabbage begins to brown along the edges and the liquid has evaporated.

4. Slice the pork chops and then serve with the cabbage.

5. Enjoy.

Nutritional information per serving: Calories 509, Fat 23g, Protein 60g, Carbs 10g

Chicken Cordon Bleu

Servings: 2

Ingredients

1 slices ham uncured

2 slices Swiss cheese

Salt and pepper to taste

1 chicken breast, boneless, skinless

Directions

1. Prepare the sous vide water bath. It should be 140F.

2. Use butter to coat the chicken breasts and then carefully place them between 2 sheets of plastic wrap. Once done, take a meat tenderizer and use it to flatten the meat.

3. Remove the meat from in between the plastic wraps and season it with some salt and pepper.

4. Arrange the Swiss cheese in the middle of each chicken breast. It should be in a single layer. Once done, place the ham on top.

5. Carefully roll up one chicken breast. You can begin rolling the chicken breast from the narrower edge and then try to form it into a jelly-like roll. Once done, roll the remaining chicken breast.

6. Place the rolled up chicken breasts in layers of plastic wraps and roll tightly. Secure the ends using twists and elastic bands. The idea is to make the wraps airtight.

7. Once done, place the prepared rolls in your sous vide bath and cook them for 1.5 hours.

8. Remove from the water and carefully remove the plastic wrap and discard it.

9. Let the chicken rest for 5-10 minutes and then slice it. Adjust the seasoning if necessary and then serve.

10. Enjoy.

Nutritional information per serving: Calories 204, Fat 11g, Protein 22g, Carbs 1g

Shrimp Scampi

Servings: 2

Ingredients

2 tablespoons parsley chopped

1 pound shrimp deveined

Salt and pepper to taste

1/8 teaspoon red chili flakes

2 tablespoons lemon juice

1/4 cup chicken broth or white wine

2 tablespoons butter

2 zucchini

Directions

1. Use a spiralizer to make the zucchini into noodle-like shapes. Once done, place the noodles on paper towels and then sprinkle some salt on them. Let them sit for about 15-30 minutes. Once done, wring out the excess moisture with dry paper towels.

2. Into a frying pan or sauté pan, melt some butter over medium heat. Once the butter has melted. Add the chicken broth, red chili flakes and lemon juice and bring the ingredients to a light boil.

3. Add the shrimp and then simmer. Once the shrimp turns pink, reduce the heat to low.

4. Taste the sauce and season with salt and pepper to your preference.

5. Add the noodles and the parsley and toss. The shrimp and noodles should be well coated in the sauce.

6. Remove and serve.

Nutritional information per serving: Calories 366, Fat 15g, Protein 49g, Carbs 7g

Mahi Mahi Bowls

Servings: 2

Ingredients

Cucumber avocado salsa:

2 tablespoons minced cilantro

2 tablespoons lime juice

2 tablespoons minced red onion

1/4 cup diced red bell pepper

1/2 cup diced cucumber

1 large avocado, diced

Macadamia crusted mahi mahi:

2 mahi mahi fillets

1/4 teaspoon salt

1/4 teaspoon onion powder

1/4 teaspoon garlic powder

1/4 teaspoon chili powder

1/4 teaspoon paprika

1/2 cup crushed macadamia nuts

Directions

1. Preheat the oven to 450 degrees F.

2. Line a baking sheet using aluminum foil or parchment.

3. Mix the spices and crushed macadamia nuts in a bowl.

4. Add the fish and press it into the mixture. Place the fish on the prepared baking sheet and bake for 10 minutes. The fish should be cooked through and golden.

5. In a bowl, add the salsa ingredients; season with salt and pepper and mix well.

6. Top the fish with salsa and serve.

Nutritional information per serving: Calories 513, Fat 41.2g, Protein 26.5g, Carbs 17.9g

Shrimp Cobb salad

Servings: 2

Ingredients

Cilantro dressing:

1/4 teaspoon sea salt

1/2 teaspoon onion powder

1/2 teaspoon ground cumin

1 clove garlic, minced

1/4 cup chopped cilantro or parsley

2 tablespoons lime juice

1/4 cup extra virgin olive oil

Cobb salad:

1 large avocado, diced

1 head Romaine lettuce

1/2 cup diced cucumber

1/2 small red onion, sliced

1/2 cup cherry tomatoes, halved

4 slices cooked bacon, chopped

2 hard-boiled eggs, quartered

8-10 large cooked shrimp/prawns

Directions

1. Carefully chop and slice the vegetables. Once done, place the dressing ingredients in a blender and pulse until smooth. This will give you a really smooth dressing. Alternatively, you can combine the dressing ingredients in a small bowl.

2. To boil the eggs, put the eggs with water in a pot and bring the water to a boil. Once it boils, turn the heat off and then cover the pot with a lid. Allow the eggs to sit for about 13 minutes. Once the time is up, transfer the eggs into a bowl that is filled with ice water. Allow them to sit for about 5 minutes.

3. In a skillet, cook the bacon for 2 minutes per side or until crispy. You can add some tablespoons of water to help cook the bacon but you don't need to add any oil.

4. Into a bowl, add the avocado, lettuce, tomato, red onion, cucumber, egg, bacon and shrimp and the dressing. Toss gently to combine and serve.

5. You can store the salad for up to 2 days in an airtight jar in the fridge if you wish.

Nutritional information per serving: Calories 671, Fat 51.8g, Protein 37.3g, Carbs 18g

Feta Summer Salad

Servings: 2

Ingredients

Dressing:

1/2 teaspoon coconut aminos or tamari sauce

1 tablespoon extra virgin olive oil

1 teaspoon lime juice

Pinch cracked black pepper, or to taste

Pinch of salt, or to taste

Salad:

1/3 cup crumbled feta

8 slices bresaola

1 tablespoon fresh mint, torn

1/4 small red onion, thinly sliced

1/2 cup cherry tomatoes, halved

1/2 large cucumber, sliced and core removed

8 scooped balls of galia melon

Directions

1. In a small bowl, combine all the dressing ingredients.

2. Peel the melon and carefully deseed it. Once done, chop the melon into bite-sized chunks.

3. Slice the cucumber lengthwise and then scoop out the seeds and discard them. Slice the cucumber.

4. In a bowl, combine the cucumber, melon, onion and tomatoes. Add the mint and dressing and toss to combine.

5. Add bresaola slices on top and then the feta.

6. Serve and enjoy. You can store the salad in your fridge for up to one day if you wish.

Nutritional information per serving: Calories 263, Fat 20g, Protein 15.1g, Carbs 7g

Keto Slaw

Servings: 2

Ingredients

Sesame seeds and green onions to garnish (if desired)

2 cloves garlic

1 tablespoon sesame oil

2 tablespoons tamari or liquid aminos

1 teaspoon vinegar

1 teaspoon chili paste, kimchi paste, or sriracha

1/2 cup macadamia nuts, chopped

4 cups shredded green cabbage

Directions

1. In a pan over medium heat, add the sesame oil, tamari, vinegar, chili paste and cabbage and toss.

2. Add in the minced garlic, cover the pan and cook for 5 minutes. The cabbage should start to wilt.

3. Stir and add in the nuts and then cook for 5 more minutes. The nuts should absorb some liquid in the pan.

4. Once done, garnish and serve.

5. Enjoy.

Nutritional information per serving: Calories 366, Fat 34.5g, Protein 5.5g, Carbs 13.4g

Salmon Salad

Servings: 2

Ingredients

Dressing:

1/2 teaspoon sea salt

1 teaspoon prepared horseradish or freshly grated horseradish

1 teaspoon Erythritol or Swerve

1 tablespoons seeded mustard

1/4 cup extra virgin olive oil

2 tablespoons fresh lemon juice

Salad ingredients:

6 Romaine lettuce leaves, torn

1 medium tomato, cut into wedges

1/4 cup fresh dill

2 tablespoons capers

2 large hard boiled eggs, quartered

150 g smoked salmon fillet, flaked

1/4 teaspoon sea salt

1 tablespoon extra virgin olive oil

1 bunch radish, trimmed

Directions

1. Preheat the oven to 410 degrees F. Meanwhile, mix the radishes, salt and olive oil and then arrange them on a lined baking tray.

2. Bake the radishes for 20-30 minutes ensuring that you turn them half way through. They should be browned and cooked through. Once done, remove them from the oven and allow them to cool a bit.

3. Prepare the dressing. Place the dressing ingredients in a small bowl or a jar and mix well to combine.

4. In the meantime, add the eggs in a saucepan and then cover them with water. Bring the water to a gentle boil. Once 7 minutes are up, remove the eggs and place them in a bowl with ice cold water. The idea is to stop the cooking process as quickly as possible.

5. Once cool, carefully peel the eggs and cut them into quarters.

6. Spread the lettuce in two plates and then sprinkle half the dill over each lettuce arrangement.

7. Divide the remaining ingredients between the two plates and then spread the remaining dill on top of each dish.

8. Serve immediately.

Nutritional information per serving: Calories 507, Fat 43.2g, Protein 22.5g, Carbs 8.8g

Chapter 4: Snacks and Desserts

Keto Sandwich

Servings: 2

Ingredients

Filling:

Salt and pepper to taste

1 teaspoon Dijon (or 2 teaspoons sugar-free ketchup)

2 slices cheddar cheese (you can use a hard cheese of your choice)

1 tablespoon butter or 2 tablespoons cream cheese

1 tablespoon ghee

2 large eggs, organic or free range

Muffins:

Pinch of salt

1/4 cup grated cheddar cheese

2 tablespoons water

2 tablespoons whipping cream (you can use coconut milk)

1 large egg, organic or free-range

1/4 teaspoon baking soda

1/4 cup flax meal

1/4 cup almond flour

Directions

1. In a small bowl, mix the dry ingredients.

2. Pour in the cream, egg and water and use a fork to mix well.

3. Carefully grate the cheese and stir it into the cream mixture.

4. Microwave the mixture for 60-90 seconds on high.

5. In the meantime, heat the ghee and fry the eggs; the whites should be opaque and the yolks should still be runny. You can fry the eggs in molds to make them fit better on the muffins. Season with a bit of salt and pepper and then remove the eggs from the heat.

6. Slice the muffins in half and then apply some butter on the insides of each half.

7. Once done, top the muffin slices with cheese, egg and some mustard and serve. You can serve with bacon and some greens if you wish. Also, you can store the muffins minus the filling for up to 3 days in airtight containers.

Nutritional information per serving: Calories 627, Fat 54.7g, Protein 25.6g, Carbs 10.2g

Mug Cake

Servings: 2

Ingredients

Mug Cake:

1/4 teaspoon vanilla extract

2 tablespoons water

2 tablespoons melted butter or avocado oil

1 large egg

Pinch salt

1/8 teaspoon cream of tartar

1/4 teaspoon cinnamon

1 teaspoon baking powder

2 table's Swerve Sweetener

2/3 cup almond flour

Cinnamon Filling/Topping:

1/2 teaspoon ground cinnamon

2 teaspoons Swerve Sweetener

Directions

1. In a bowl, gently whisk together the cinnamon and sweetener to make the filling. Set aside.

2. In another bowl, mix the baking powder, sweetener, almond flour, cream of tartar, salt and cinnamon.

3. Once done, add the egg, water, oil or butter and vanilla extract; stir the ingredients well to combine.

4. Portion half the mixture into two coffee mugs and then add the topping or filling into each mug. Make sure you divide the filling evenly. Once done, portion the remaining half batter into two and use each portion to top the filling.

5. Microwave the ingredients for 1 minute on high. The mug cakes should be cooked through and puffed.

6. Serve immediately. You can serve with milk or cream if you wish.

Nutritional information per serving: Calories 323, Fat 29.38g, Protein 8.16g, Carbs 9.50g

English Muffins

Servings: 2

Ingredients

1/8 teaspoon salt

1/4 teaspoon baking powder

1 tablespoon coconut flour

1 egg at room temperature

1 1/2 tablespoons almond butter

1 1/2 teaspoons coconut oil, softened

Directions

1. In a microwave safe cup, mix the egg, almond butter and coconut oil, and stir well.

2. Add the baking powder, salt and coconut flour and stir well to incorporate.

3. Once done, microwave for 60 to 90 seconds on high.

4. Carefully remove the muffin and slice it in half.

5. Serve immediately while still warm.

Nutritional information per serving: Calories 146, Fat 12g, Protein 5g, Carbs 4g

Asparagus Fries

Servings: 2

Ingredients

1 tablespoon roasted red pepper, finely chopped

3 tablespoons mayonnaise

2 large eggs

½ teaspoon smoked paprika

¼ cup almond flour

½ teaspoon garlic powder

2 tablespoons parsley, chopped

½ cup Parmesan cheese, shredded

10 medium asparagus spears

Directions

1. Preheat the oven to 425 degrees F.

2. Carefully wash and rinse the asparagus spears. In your food processor, add the parsley, garlic powder and shredded parmesan cheese and then pulse until fine.

3. Add the almond flour into the food processor and then pulse again to incorporate. Once done, place the mixture in a shallow dish and then proceed to stir in the smoked paprika.

4. In another bowl, thoroughly beat two eggs until frothy. This will help them adhere to the asparagus.

5. Hold the end of the asparagus spears and carefully dip each piece into the egg mixture.

6. Once done, hold the spears near the bowl with the parmesan flour mixture and then carefully sprinkle the mixture onto the spears and coat them well. Do not place the spears directly into the flour mix as this will cause them to become lumpy.

7. Once all the spears are coated, arrange them tightly on a baking sheet and then spread the leftover parmesan mixture on top.

8. Bake the asparagus fries for 10 minutes. The asparagus should be slightly tender.

9. In a small bowl, combine the mayonnaise and roasted red pepper. Make sure the red pepper is finely chopped first to make it easier to incorporate. Once done, place the dip

in the refrigerator and allow it to chill. When you're ready to serve, stir the dip well.

10. Serve the asparagus fries with the dip.

11. Enjoy.

Nutritional information per serving: Calories 453.65, Fat 33.43g, Protein 19.14g, Carbs 5.51g

Portobello Mushroom Fries

Servings: 2

Ingredients

1 tablespoon dried chives, to garnish

1/4 cup shredded cheddar cheese

3 strips bacon

1 large egg, beaten

1/4 teaspoon cayenne pepper

1/2 teaspoon smoked paprika

1/2 teaspoon garlic powder

1/2 cup shredded Parmesan cheese

2 large Portobello mushroom caps

Directions

1. Preheat the oven to 425 degrees F and then spray a baking sheet with non-stick spray or line with foil.

2. Cut the mushrooms into thick strips. They should be about 1/4 inches thick. You can slice the ends off such that the strips resemble a French fry.

3. Into a food processor, pulse together the seasonings and the parmesan cheese and then transfer the mixture to a shallow dish or bowl.

4. In another bowl, beat the egg and then dip the mushroom slices in the egg. Make sure they are coated well.

5. Once done, roll the slices in the parmesan mixture and then arrange them on the prepared baking sheet. Roast the mushroom fries for 10 minutes.

6. In the meantime, place a pan over medium heat and add the bacon strips. Cook until crisp. Once done, remove from the heat and let them cool. Dice or crumble using a knife.

7. Once the fries are done, remove them from the oven and spread the crumbled bacon and shredded cheese on top. Bake the mixture for 5 more minutes until it melts

8. Once the fries are ready, serve with dried chives.

Nutritional information per serving: Calories 280, Fat 18.97g, Protein 21.82g, Carbs 5.9g

Keto Poke

Servings: 2

Ingredients

1/4 ruby red grapefruit

1 teaspoon sea salt

1/4 cup pili nuts

1 tablespoon sesame seeds

2 tablespoons sesame oil

1/2 Hass avocado

5 sprigs cilantro or Italian parsley (about 1/4 cup chopped)

1 tablespoon coconut aminos

8oz. Yellow Fin Tuna (Ahi Tuna) Fillet

Directions

1. Slice the tuna into 1/4 inch cubes and then place the cubes in a bowl.

2. In the bowl, add the coconut aminos, salt and sesame oil. Toss gently to coat.

3. Slice the grapefruit into sections and then add the pieces into the bowl.

4. Once done, mince the cilantro and spread it over the ingredients in the bowl.

5. Dice the avocado and chop the pili nuts and add them to the bowl.

6. Toss the ingredients to mix everything.

7. Portion into two and spread some sesame seeds on top.

8. Serve and enjoy.

Nutritional information per serving: Calories 445, Fat 33g, Protein 39g, Carbs 10g

Chocolate Mug Cake

Servings: 2

Ingredients

Pinch kosher salt

1/2 teaspoon baking powder

2 teaspoons coconut flour

1 tablespoon golden flaxseed meal or psyllium husk, finely ground

2 tablespoons almond flour

1 egg

2-3 tablespoons xylitol or erythritol

1 1/2 tablespoons cocoa powder

2 tablespoons unsalted grass-fed butter

Directions

1. In a microwave safe bowl, melt the butter. Once melted, add the sweetener and cocoa and whisk until well combined. If you are using erythritol, the batter will likely be very thick. As such, you need to whisk well.

109

2. Add the egg and continue to whisk until smooth, and then add the remaining ingredients and whisk to combine. Once done, spoon the mixture into your mug. The mixture tends to be quite thick.

3. In your microwave, add a paper towel. Once done, place the mug on top of the paper towel in order to trap any overflowing batter.

4. Cook for 70-90 seconds on high.

5. Once ready, allow the mug cake to cool and then serve.

Nutritional information per serving: Calories 219, Fat 17g, Protein 6g, Carbs 7.5g

Chapter 5: Keto Beverages

Lemon Ginger Green Juice

Servings: 2

Ingredients

1 teaspoon of erythritol

1 Tablespoon of fresh ginger, peeled and roughly diced

Generous handful mint leaves

2 tablespoons of lemon juice

5 stalks of trimmed celery, roughly chopped

5.3 oz. of kale, roughly chopped

Directions

1. Place the ingredients minus the sweetener into your juicer. Once done, switch on the juicer and process until you have the juice.

2. Discard the pulp or us it in your stews.

3. Add the sweetener and stir to mix in.

4. Top the juice with ice if you wish.

5. Enjoy.

Nutritional information per serving: Calories 51, Fat 0g, Protein 3g, Carbs 11g

Blueberry Ginger Smoothie

Servings: 2

Ingredients

Stevia, to taste

1 teaspoon MCT oil

3 slices of ginger

1 cup coconut milk (from cartons, unsweetened)

1/2 cup coconut yogurt

15 blueberries

Directions

1. Place the ingredients into a blender, and process until smooth.

2. Serve.

Nutritional information per serving: Calories 168, Fat 15g, Protein 4g, Carbs 5g

Cucumber Green Tea Smoothie

Servings: 2

Ingredients

1/2 cup ice

1/2 teaspoon liquid stevia

1 teaspoon lemon juice

2 ounces ripe avocado

1 cup sliced cucumber

2 teaspoon Match Green Tea powder

8 ounces water

Directions

1. Into a blender, add the green tea and water. Whirl the ingredients to combine.

2. Once done, add the other ingredients and then pulse on high.

3. Taste the smoothie and adjust the sweetener to your desired level of sweetness.

4. Drink immediately or store in the fridge for later.

5. Enjoy.

Nutritional information per serving: Calories 69, Fat 4.6g, Protein 2g, Carbs 6.8g

Almond Butter Smoothie

Servings: 2

Ingredients

1 cup ice

1/2 medium hass avocado

2 tablespoons almond butter

Pinch pink sea salt

1/2 teaspoon vanilla extract

3 tablespoons erythritol granular

2 tablespoons cacao powder

3/4 cup water

1/2 cup canned coconut milk, full fat or heavy cream

Directions

1. Add the canned coconut milk and water into the blender, before adding the remaining ingredients and pulse to combine.

2. Once done, pour the smoothies in 2 glasses and serve.

3. Enjoy.

Nutritional information per serving: Calories 328, Fat 30g, Protein 7g, Carbs 15g

Tasty Smoothie

Servings: 2

Ingredients

2 cups ice cubes

1 scoop low carb protein powder vanilla

2 tablespoons walnuts or any type of low carb nut

2 tablespoons coconut shredded + unsweetened

3/4 cup blackberries

1/2 cup low carb milk such as coconut milk

Hemp Seeds topping, optional

Directions

1. Add the ingredients into the blender and blend to your desired consistency.

2. Divide between two glasses and serve. You can top with some ice cubes if you wish.

3. Enjoy.

Nutritional information per serving: Calories 185, Fat 11g, Protein 13g, Carbs 8g

Chocolate Berry Smoothie

Servings: 2

Ingredients

3/4 cup ice cubes

3/4 cup frozen mixed berries such as raspberries, strawberries, and blueberries

1/2 cup water

1/4 cup heavy whipping cream

3/4 teaspoon pure vanilla extract

1 pinch salt

2 (1g) packets stevia/erythritol blend

1 1/2 tablespoons unsweetened cocoa powder

2 tablespoons pecans or almonds

1/2 medium-sized avocado

Optional Toppings:

Shaved stevia-sweetened chocolate

Fresh or frozen berries

Directions

1. Halve the avocado and peel it and then place all the smoothie ingredients except the ice in your blender and then pulse to your desired level of smoothness.

2. Add in the ice cubes and continue to pulse until incorporated.

3. Pour the smoothie into two glasses and serve immediately.

4. Enjoy.

Nutritional information per serving: Calories 294, Fat 26g, Protein 3g, Carbs 15g

Strawberry and Almond Butter Smoothie

Servings: 2

Ingredients

1 ½ cups almond milk

1 scoop dairy free vanilla protein powder (about 30g)

2 tablespoons almond butter

1 cup frozen mixed berries

Directions

1. Dump the ingredients in a blender.

2. Pulse until you get a smooth and creamy consistency.

3. Pour into glasses and serve immediately.

Nutritional information per serving: Calories 140, Fat 4g, Protein 0g, Carbs 11g

Keto Shake

Servings: 2

Ingredients

12–16 ice cubes

1/4 teaspoon salt

1/4 teaspoon almond extract

30 drops liquid stevia

1 teaspoon cinnamon

4 tablespoons golden flax meal

4 tablespoons almond butter

2 scoop collagen peptides

3 cups unsweetened nut milk

Directions

1. Place the ingredients in a blender and blend until smooth. This should take about 30 seconds.

2. Serve immediately.

Nutritional information per serving: Calories 326, Fat 27g, Protein 19g, Carbs 11g

Strawberry Avocado Smoothie

Servings: 2

Ingredients

1/2 cup ice more or less

2 stevia packets

1 tablespoon lime juice

1 1/2 cups coconut milk

1 medium avocado

2/3 cup frozen strawberries

Directions

1. Pour all the ingredients into a blender and pulse until smooth and serve.

Nutritional information per serving: Calories 165, Fat 14g, Protein 2g, Carbs 11g

Raspberry Avocado Smoothie

Servings: 2

Ingredients

1/2 cup frozen unsweetened raspberries

1/8 teaspoon liquid stevia extract

2-3 tablespoons lemon juice

1 1/3 cups water

1 ripe avocado peeled and pit removed

Directions

1. Place the frozen raspberries, sweetener, lemon juice and water in your blender and blend until smooth.

2. Serve.

Nutritional information per serving: Calories 227, Fat 20g, Protein 2.5g, Carbs 12.8g

Keto Peach Tea

Servings: 2

Ingredients

6-8 ice cubes

1 scoop Perfect Keto Peach Exogenous Ketones

¼ teaspoon stevia

1 teaspoon vanilla extract

½ cup heavy cream

1 cup hot water

1 organic oolong tea bag

Directions

1. Prepare hot water and steep the tea for about 4 minutes.

2. Once done, carefully remove the tea bag and discard it. Pour the tea into a blender and then add the remaining ingredients but don't add the ice. Blend well to combine.

3. Once well-combined, pour the ice into two glasses.

4. Add the tea into each glass and swirl gently.

5. Enjoy.

Nutritional information per serving: Calories 210, Fat 24g, Protein 0g, Carbs 0g

Coconut Milk Latte

Servings: 2

Ingredients

Dash of cinnamon, optional

1/2 cup coconut cream or full-fat coconut milk

3 cups prepared hot coffee

Directions

1. Into a blender, add the coconut milk and coffee.

2. Blend the mixture for 1 minute on medium-high. The coconut milk should be completely incorporated.

3. Pour some ice in two mugs and then add the coconut milk latte. You can add more coconut milk if you wish.

4. Serve and enjoy.

Nutritional information per serving: Calories 114, Fat 12g, Protein 1g, Carbs 1g

Cacao Coffee

Servings: 2

Ingredients

Cinnamon powder (just a pinch)

Coconut oil melted, just a splash

1/2 teaspoon gelatin

Boiling water

1 cup Cacao nibs

Directions

1. Preheat the oven to 350 degrees F.

2. Arrange the cacao nibs on a baking sheet in a thin layer.

3. Once done, put the baking sheet in your oven and roast for 15-18 minutes.

4. Remove the cacao nibs from the oven and let them cool. Once they've cooled, store them in an airtight container.

5. In order to prepare cacao coffee, you'll need 1 cup of boiling water per tablespoon of the cacao nibs. Start by placing the cacao nubs in the coffee grinder and pulse

well. You can pulse four times each 2 seconds until you get a powder.

6. Once done, remove the powder and add it to the French press before adding the boiling water. Allow the mixture to steep for about 5-8 minutes.

7. In a cup, add a splash of cold water and the gelatin and stir well using a spoon.

8. Add in coconut oil, cinnamon and cacao coffee into the cup and mix well to combine.

9. Serve immediately.

Nutritional information per serving: Calories 335, Fat 28g, Protein 8g, Carbs 10g

Keto Brownie Shake

Servings: 2

Ingredients

1–2 cups crushed ice

Erythritol or stevia, to taste

20 fl oz. unsweetened almond milk

2 tablespoons hot water

3 tablespoons unsweetened cacao powder

1 tablespoon chopped walnuts of a few slices of avocado (for garnish)

Directions

1. In a large bowl, mix the cacao powder and a bit of hot water. Make sure the cacao powder dissolves well before adding the almond milk.

2. Mix the ingredients well and then add the sweetener. Taste and adjust the sweetener if necessary.

3. Cover the bowl and chill in the fridge.

4. Place a little crushed ice in two glasses and then top the glasses with the chocolate drink.

5. Garnish the drinks with chopped walnuts and serve.

6. Enjoy.

Nutritional information per serving: Calories 112, Fat 8g, Protein 5g, carbs 7g

Avocado Smoothie

Servings: 2

Ingredients

1 teaspoon unsweetened shredded coconut, for garnish

1 teaspoon MCT oil

1 tablespoon lime juice

1/2 cup coconut milk (unsweetened, from a carton)

1 large avocado, de-stoned

Directions

1. Slice the avocado in half lengthwise and then discard the seed.

2. Peel and cube the avocado and then place all the ingredients in the blender and blend well.

3. Pour into glasses and enjoy.

Nutritional information per serving: Calories 227, Fat 19g, Protein 7g, Carbs 10g

Strawberry Bourbon

Servings: 2

Ingredients

Pinch of ground black pepper

2 ounce fresh lemon juice

4 ounces bourbon

2 teaspoon powdered erythritol

6 basil leaves

6 strawberries, hulled and sliced

Directions

1. In a glass, add some ice.

2. In a cocktail shaker, combine the basil, erythritol, bourbon and strawberries and then shake. The basil and strawberries should be crushed. This will release their juices.

3. Once done, add the pepper and lemon juice and then add some ice to the cocktail shaker and shake well.

4. Strain the mixture and place it in the glass.

5. Garnish with basil and a strawberry slice and serve.

6. Enjoy.

Nutritional information per serving: Calories 159, Fat 0.4g, Protein 0.5g, Carbs 3.5g

Tart Cranberry Cooler

Servings: 2

Ingredients

4 ounces prosecco

4 lime wedges, extra for garnish

4 ounces dry gin

4 teaspoons powdered erythritol, more to taste

20 fresh cranberries, extra for garnish

Directions

1. Fill a large glass with some ice.

2. In a cocktail shaker, combine the gin, lime juice, lime wedges, cranberries, erythritol and gin. Muddle the ingredients until the cranberries and limes are crushed; thus, releasing their juices.

3. Strain the mixture and add it to the glass with ice.

4. Top the cocktail with prosecco and then garnish with a lime wedge and cranberries.

5. Serve and enjoy.

Nutritional information per serving: Calories 203, Fat 0g, Protein 0g, Carbs 4g

Blueberry Mojito

Servings: 2

Ingredients

10 blueberries, for garnish

Club soda

8 fresh mint leaves

2 teaspoon powdered erythritol, more to taste

Juice of 1 lime

4 ounces white rum

Directions

1. Lightly muddle the lime juice, erythritol, rum and mint leaves.

2. Pour the mixture over ice and then top with the club soda, and serve.

3. You can garnish with blueberries if your wish.

Nutritional information per serving: Calories 90, Fat 0g, Protein 0g, Carbs 4g

Keto Gin Cocktail

Servings: 2

Ingredients

Club soda

2 teaspoon powdered erythritol, more to taste

1 ounce fresh lime juice

4 ounces dry gin

10 fresh mint leaves

8 blueberries

Directions

1. In a cocktail shaker, add the mint and blueberries. Once done, muddle the ingredients until they release their juices.

2. Add the lime juice, erythritol, gin and ice. Place the cap and shake well.

3. Strain the mixture and pour into glasses and then top with the club soda.

4. Serve. You can garnish with fresh mint if you wish.

Nutritional information per serving: Calories 139, Fat 0.1g, Protein 0.2g, Carbs 2.9g

Conclusion

We have come to the end of the book. Thank you for reading and congratulations for reading until the end.

Finally, I would like to ask you for a favour. Can you please leave a review for this book? I will greatly appreciate that.

Thank you and Good Luck!

Thank You

My Other Books

If you love this book, I have other ketogenic diet books that may interest you.

Keto Bread

https://www.amazon.com/Keto-Bread-Flatbread-Tortillas-Cornbread-ebook/dp/B07S16MNGM/ref=sr_1_64?keywords=Keto+bread&qid=1565622803&s=digital-text&sr=1-64

Keto Fat Bombs

https://www.amazon.com/Keto-Fat-Bombs-Optimal-Ketosis-ebook/dp/B07RVPKGL7/ref=sr_1_1?keywords=Keto+fat+bombs%3A+over+70+sweet+and+savory&qid=1565623307&s=digital-text&sr=1-1

Keto Meal Plan

https://www.amazon.com/Keto-Meal-Plan-Ketogenic-Delicious-

ebook/dp/B07R4JSC2B/ref=sr_1_1?keywords=keto+meal+
plan%3A+90+day+ketogenic&qid=1565623382&s=digital-
text&sr=1-1

The Simple 5 Ingredient Keto Cookbook

https://www.amazon.com/Simple-Ingredient-Keto-
Cookbook-Ingredients-
ebook/dp/B07R6BH3JK/ref=sr_1_8?keywords=the+simple
+5+ingredient+keto+cookbook&qid=1565623477&s=digital-
text&sr=1-8

Keto Air fryer Recipes

https://www.amazon.com/dp/B07WFQTXQN

Made in the USA
Thornton, CO
08/08/24 00:24:43

a206e8c9-6738-4003-8106-644f707959e7R01